Tic Talk: My Hilarious Journey with Tourette's"

Can't you just stop it?

Alina White

To my beloved captors,

Thank you for giving me the gift of Tourette's, without which I wouldn't be able to write this hilarious and informative book. Your tireless dedication to making me twitch and shout at the most inappropriate times has truly paid off.

Mom and Dad, your support has been invaluable in helping me navigate this world with Tourette's. Who needs polite small talk at church when you can let loose with some colorful language, right? And thanks, Dad, for turning my tics into a job interview superpower. If a potential employer can't handle a little twitching and shaking, then they clearly can't handle the high-pressure work environment that comes with hiring a ticker like me.

But let's not forget all the other ways you've helped me out. Mom, your obsession with hand-washing has really added to my collection of tics. Every time I see a sink now, I can't help but think of you and your endless reminders. But hey, at least my hands are clean enough to perform surgery, even if my brain is still a little wonky. And Dad, your "jump out and scare Alina" has taught me to always be on my toes and ready for anything. Who needs a gym membership when you've got a dad who can make you jump a foot in the air?

In all seriousness though, I couldn't have made it this far without your love and support. You've always been there to laugh with me when things get tough, and to remind me that my tics are nothing to be ashamed of. So here's to you, Mom and Dad, for being the best parents a ticker could ask for.

So here's to you, Mom and Dad, the real MVPs of Tic Talk. I hope this book makes you proud, or at least makes you laugh so hard you forget about all the times I accidentally kicked you in the shins.

With love and tics,
Alina

Table of contents:

Can't you just stop it?

Can't you just stop it?

A One-Woman Circus Act

Well, hello there! My name is Alina, and I'm excited to share my journey through life with Tourette's in this book. I mean, who doesn't want to read about a lovely lady with a potty mouth and an uncontrollable urge to twitch and shout, am I right?

So, let me start by saying that having Tourette's is not all bad. Sure, I may look like a freakshow to some, but I like to think of myself as a one-woman circus act. I mean, who needs acrobats and clowns when you have me around, right?

In this book, I'm going to take you through my Tourette's journey, from the moment I first started ticking to my struggles in the workplace. But don't worry, I won't bore you with medical jargon and scientific explanations. I'll leave that to the doctors and scientists who get paid the big bucks.

Instead, I'm going to share with you the joys of twitching and shouting, the awkward moments in school, and the challenges of dating with Tourette's. Spoiler alert: it's not easy, folks. But hey, at least I have an excuse for being single, right?

I'll also be sharing some of my tried-and-failed coping mechanisms, like meditation and deep breathing. Who needs Zen when you can just scream obscenities at the top of your lungs? Trust me, it's much more cathartic.

And let's not forget about the humor in tics. Yes, I know it sounds crazy, but sometimes I can't help but laugh at myself when I'm ticking like a maniac in public. It's like my own personal comedy show.

But unfortunately, not everyone sees the humor in it. In fact, there's still a lot of stigma surrounding Tourette's. Some people still think we're possessed by the devil or just plain crazy. But don't worry, I'll teach you how to convince people that you're not a lunatic.

So, get ready to laugh, cry, and cringe as I take you on a journey through life with Tourette's. And who knows, maybe by the end of this book, you'll be twitching and shouting right alongside me.

Welcome to the Freak Show: My Tourette's Journey Begins

Buckle up and get ready for a wild ride because in this chapter, I'm going to take you back to the beginning of my Tourette's journey. It's not always rainbows and unicorns, but I promise it'll be entertaining. From the initial confusion and shock of the diagnosis to discovering the joy of tics, this is where it all began. So, come along for the ride and let's see where this adventure takes us.

Why Fit In When You Can Stand Out?

When I was a mere child, something very strange started happening to me. My body would move uncontrollably, and I would make weird noises that would make even the weirdest people go, "What the hell is wrong with you?" But being a kid, I didn't pay much attention to it. I mean, who cares, right? As long as I could keep playing with my toys and get my sugar fix, what else mattered?

But soon enough, it became apparent that something was very off about me. I was the kid who would randomly shout out curse words during math class, the one who would make bizarre facial expressions during family gatherings, and the one who would flail my arms around like a demented penguin on the playground. It was like I was cursed with an inner demon that just couldn't be contained.

At first, it was tough. I mean, who wants to be the kid who can't control their own body? But then I realized something: if I couldn't beat my tics, I might as well join them. I started to embrace my weirdness, letting my body do whatever the hell it wanted to do. And let me tell you, it was like a goddamn carnival in there.

People would stare at me, of course, wondering what the hell was wrong with this strange creature flapping around

Can't you just stop it?

like a drunken bird. But I didn't care. I was a walking, talking freak show, and damn it, I was proud of it. It was like I had my own secret superpower that nobody else knew about, and it was freaking awesome.

It's Not a Tumor!

As I sat there contemplating my newfound uniqueness, I could hear my parents in the next room talking about what to do with me now that I had been diagnosed with Tourette's. I could hear my dad saying, "Well, it's not a tumor, so I guess that's a relief." I rolled my eyes.

My mom, on the other hand, was trying to be positive, as usual. "Oh, she's just unique, and that's something to be proud of!" I could practically hear the eye roll in her voice, too. Unique? More like a freak show, but I appreciate the effort, Mom.

But bless their hearts, they never gave up. They tried all sorts of things to help me manage my tics, from meditation to medication. It was almost cute how they tried to make light of the situation, like when my dad would say things like, "At least we don't have to worry about her lying to us!" or my mom would exclaim, "Look at her go! She could be a drummer!" I appreciated the effort, even if it did make me want to roll my eyes so hard they would pop out of my head.

I have to give them credit, though. They never stopped trying to understand what I was going through. They read books on Tourette's, watched documentaries, and went to support groups for families with tic disorders. I guess it made them feel better to know that they weren't the only ones dealing with a child who sounded like a Tourette's-afflicted pirate.

I have to say that my parents handled my Tourette's with as much grace and humor as anyone could expect. They never made me feel like a freak or a burden, even when I was at my worst. And honestly, that's all I could have asked for.

Hey, Look at Me!

As I learned more about Tourette's, I discovered that it wasn't all bad. In fact, there was something kind of liberating about being able to make weird noises and movements without worrying about what other people thought. I started experimenting with different tics, seeing what kind of reactions I could get out of people. My favorite was a high-pitched squeak that sounded like a cartoon mouse. It always made people do a double-take.

One time, I was at a family gathering and feeling self-conscious about my tics. I was trying to suppress them as much as possible, but it was like trying to hold in a fart in a quiet room. Suddenly, my leg jerked out and kicked my aunt's cat. The cat screeched and ran away as my aunt gave me the stink eye.

The room went quiet as everyone glared at me. They were waiting for me to freak out or burst into tears or something. But then I started to laugh. I couldn't help it. It was like my tic had broken the tension in the room, and suddenly everyone was laughing too. It was one of those moments where I felt like I was part of something bigger than myself, like my weirdness was actually bringing people together.

After that, I just let my tics fly. I was like a human pinball machine, bouncing around the room and knocking things over. It was like a game of "Tourette's Bingo" and everyone was having a blast. Sure, I got some weird looks and a few people probably thought I was possessed, but hey, at least I was entertaining.

Looking back, I'm glad I didn't try to suppress my tics that day. If I had, I would have missed out on all the laughs and fun. Who knew that being a little "unique" could bring so much joy to others?

Tics, Schmics: The Joy of Twitching and Shouting

Ah, tics. The involuntary movements and vocalizations that make you look like you're auditioning for a one-person avant-garde performance piece. It's like having your own little sideshow act, and you never know what weird and wonderful things your body will do next. So come one, come all, and step right up to experience the joy of twitching and shouting with me.

Can't you just stop it?

Tic, Tic, Boom!

Tics, those uncontrollable, irresistible movements or sounds that we Touretters know all too well. But did you know that there are countless types of tics, each with their own unique flair? Allow me to introduce you to some of my personal favorites.

First up, we have the classic motor tics, like head-jerking, eye-blinking, and shoulder-shrugging. They're like the greatest hits of tics, the ones everyone knows and loves. But why stop there when you can get creative? How about flapping your arms like a bird, or doing a full-body shimmy like you're auditioning for a dance troupe? Trust me, the possibilities are endless.

And let's not forget about the vocal tics. Who needs to talk normally when you can add in a few "woofs" or "meows" for good measure? Or maybe you're more of a "boop" or "beep" kind of person? Whatever your preference, vocal tics are a great way to spice up any conversation.

To Shout or Not to Shout?

One of the greatest challenges of having Tourette's is learning to control those pesky tics when necessary. Sure, it's all fun and games when you're alone in your room, but what about when you're in a public place or trying to have a serious conversation? That's when things get tricky.

For me, the hardest part has always been the shouting tics. There's nothing quite like suddenly blurting out an expletive in the middle of a crowded room to make you feel like a complete and utter jackass. So, I've developed a few strategies over the years to try to keep those impulses in check.

First and foremost, there's the old standby of biting my tongue. Literally. It's not exactly pleasant, but it's effective in a pinch. Then there's the classic distraction technique of squeezing a stress ball or fidgeting with something in my hands. And of course, there's always the tried-and-true method of just walking away from the situation altogether.

But let's be real here, sometimes the tics are just too strong to resist. In those moments, all you can do is own it and hope for the best. Apologize profusely, make a self-deprecating joke, and move on. After all, life is too short to worry about what other people think.

Life's Too Short to Suppress Tics

Speaking of not worrying about what other people think, let's talk about the pure, unadulterated joy of letting those tics fly.

Can't you just stop it?

There's nothing quite like the feeling of giving in to that urge and just letting your body do its thing.

For me, it's like a physical release, a way to let out all the pent-up energy and frustration that builds up over time. Sure, it might look a little weird to outsiders, but who cares? It feels amazing.

And you know what? Sometimes, those tics can even be a source of entertainment for others. I've lost count of how many times I've made a room full of people laugh with a well-timed "quack" or "honk." It's like being a one-person comedy show, and who wouldn't love that?

So, fellow Touretters, I say embrace your tics. Let them out, let them be weird, and let them bring a little joy into your life. Life's too short to suppress the things that make us unique, after all.

Can't you just stop it?

I'm Not Crazy, I'm Just Tourettesy: The Diagnosis and What It Really Means

Welcome to the world of Tourette's, where you can't control your movements, your words, or your awkward social encounters. But hey, at least you have an excuse, right? In this chapter, we'll explore the diagnosis of Tourette's and what it really means to have this wacky condition.

Can't you just stop it?

It's Not Me, It's You

When people hear the word "Tourette's," they automatically think of that one kid from the movie who couldn't stop screaming out obscenities. But let me tell you, as someone with Tourette's, it's not all fun and games.

Sure, my tics may seem entertaining to you, but to me, they're just a daily inconvenience that I have to deal with. And don't even get me started on the looks and stares I get from strangers when I'm in the middle of a tic. It's like they've never seen someone flapping their arms like a bird or barking like a dog before.

But here's the thing, my tics are just a part of who I am. I've had them since I was a kid, and they've become so normal to me that I barely even notice them anymore. It's like having a third arm - yeah, it's strange, but you learn to live with it.

Now, I know what you're thinking. "Can't you just stop?" "Can't you control it?" Let me tell you, it's not that simple. It's like trying to hold your breath underwater for hours on end - eventually, your body is going to do what it needs to do. And in my case, that means ticking.

And don't even get me started on the myths surrounding Tourette's. No, I'm not possessed by a demon, and no, I can't just "pray it away." Trust me, I've tried. It's a neurological condition, not a spiritual one.

Can't you just stop it?

Don't get me wrong, the swearing tics do happen. But they're not the norm, and they're not the only thing that Tourette's is about. For me, it's more about the physical tics - the sudden jerks, the weird facial expressions, the little noises that I make without even realizing it.

It's like having a tiny monster inside me, constantly poking and prodding me to move or make a sound. And if I don't do it, if I try to hold back or suppress the tics, it's like the monster gets even more agitated and starts throwing a tantrum. So yeah, it's kind of like being possessed by a demon, I guess. But it's not like I chose to be possessed, you know? It's just something that happened to me, like getting struck by lightning or winning the lottery.

And the thing is, as weird and uncomfortable as the tics can be, they're also kind of hilarious. I mean, have you ever seen someone suddenly jerk their head to the side or flap their arms like a bird? It's like a scene straight out of a cartoon. And when it's happening to me, I can't help but laugh. It's either that or cry, and I'd much rather laugh.

Of course, not everyone sees the humor in it. Some people get freaked out or offended by my tics, like I'm some kind of contagious disease or public menace. And then there are the people who think it's okay to make fun of me, to mimic my tics or call me names. To those people, I have one thing to say: really? You're going to stoop that low? You're going to

Can't you just stop it?

mock someone for something they have no control over, just to get a cheap laugh? That's just sad.

But hey, I'm not going to let those people bring me down. I've got my tiny monster, my secret superpower, and I'm not afraid to use it. So if you see me suddenly jerking my head to the side or flapping my arms like a bird, don't be alarmed. It's just me, embracing my inner freak and living my best life

It's Not a Choice, It's a Superpower

Sure, there are plenty of downsides to having Tourette's, like feeling like a circus act or having people stare at you like you're some sort of alien. But sometimes you just have to laugh it off and embrace the weirdness. And trust me, there's a lot of weirdness to embrace.

I mean, who else gets to have a built-in excuse for all their strange behavior? Forgot someone's name? Tic attack. Accidentally spilled coffee on your coworker's shirt? Tic attack. Want to get out of a boring conversation? Tic attack. It's like having a get-out-of-jail-free card for social interactions.

And let's not forget the never-ending entertainment value of Tourette's. With a constantly evolving repertoire of tics, life is never boring. It's like playing a never-ending game of charades, but instead of acting out words, your body just decides to do it for you.

Who Needs a Personality When You Have Tics?

It's no secret that Tourette's can be a major part of one's identity, for better or for worse. But where do the tics end and the "real you" begin? It's a complicated question that doesn't have an easy answer. We'll delve into the complexities of Tourette's and identity, including how to navigate relationships, careers, and everyday life with this condition.

One time, I was at a friend's birthday party and I accidentally shouted "banana hammock!" in the middle of the Happy Birthday song. My friend's mom gave me a disapproving look, but I just explained, "Hey, it's not my fault, it's the Tourette's talking!" Needless to say, I was the life of the party.

Another time, I was in class and couldn't stop twitching my eyebrows. My teacher asked me if I needed to use the restroom and I replied, "Nope, just my Tourette's having a party on my face!" I didn't get in trouble, but at least I made everyone laugh. Who needs good grades when you've got a great sense of humor?

Can't you just stop it?

The Early Years: Making Friends and Influencing People with My Tics

Welcome to my childhood, where my Tourette's turned me into a real-life version of that whack-a-mole game. I mean, sure, my parents were concerned about my well-being and my teachers were worried about my disruptive behavior in class. But little did they know, I was just honing my skills as a future stand-up comedian. I had a whole arsenal of tics to choose from: head jerks, eye blinks, throat clears, and even the occasional animal noise. It was like my body was a jukebox and I could play any song I wanted.

Of course, there were some downsides to this whole Tourette's thing. Like the time I accidentally barked during a moment of silence in a school assembly. Or the time I yelled "penis" in the middle of a crowded mall. But hey, nobody's perfect. And let's be real, those moments were pretty damn funny.

I quickly learned that humor was my greatest weapon against the bullies and the skeptics. If I could make them laugh, they were less likely to mock me. And if they did, well, I had plenty of comebacks at the ready. "At least my tics are more interesting than your personality!" or "Hey, at least I have a medical excuse for being weird!"

It wasn't all laughs and giggles, though. There were times when I felt like a freak, like I would never be able to fit in with the "normal" kids. But then I realized, why would I want to be normal? Being different was what made me special. And if people couldn't accept that, then they weren't worth my time.

Of course, it wasn't all fun and games. I had to navigate the tricky terrain of making and keeping friends, all while trying to explain to them that no, I'm not possessed by a demon, I just have Tourette's. It was like being a one-person circus, with my tics as the star attraction.

The Kids Are Alright (Until They're Not)

Being a young ticker was like being trapped in a never-ending game show where the host was a sadistic jerk. He'd make you shout out embarrassing words and twitch like a marionette with a broken string. And no matter how hard you tried to resist, you were always forced to play along. It was like living in a nightmare version of "Whose Line Is It Anyway?" where the points didn't matter and the only prize was a lifetime supply of tics.

I quickly learned that kids can be brutal. They would imitate my tics and make fun of me until I felt like I was living in a bad sitcom. But, hey, at least I always had a witty comeback ready to go. It's hard to make fun of someone when they're screaming "pickle juice" in your face.

One time, in the middle of class, my tics got the best of me and I let out a loud screech that sounded like a cross between a dying cat and a tea kettle. Everyone turned to look at me, and I could feel my face turning red with embarrassment. But then, a miracle happened. My best friend Lisa stood up and let out an even louder screech, followed by a round of applause from the class. It was like we were in a competition to see who could make the most noise, and I was determined to win.

Another time, during a school assembly, I couldn't stop twitching my nose like a bunny on crack. Everyone was

Can't you just stop it?

staring at me, but I didn't care. I was in my own world, twitching away. And then, the principal started talking about bullying and how we should all treat each other with kindness and respect. I couldn't help but laugh out loud. I mean, the irony was just too much.

But not all of my childhood memories with Tourette's were funny. Some were downright terrifying. Like the time I was walking home from school and a group of older kids started following me, taunting me, and throwing things at me. I was terrified, but my tics kicked in and I started shouting and flailing my arms like a maniac. I must have looked insane because they quickly backed off and ran away. That's when I realized the true power of my Tourette's - it could scare away even the toughest bullies.

Looking back, I realize that my Tourette's was both a blessing and a curse. It made me stand out in a crowd, which was both good and bad. But most importantly, it taught me to embrace my quirks and not give a damn about what other people thought. Because at the end of the day, I was the one with the most interesting stories to tell.

The Art of Scaring Friends and Family

As I got older, I started to realize that my tics could be more than just a source of embarrassment. They could be downright hilarious. It's amazing how many people will laugh at your tics when you present them as a joke instead of a disability. I quickly became the life of the party, using my tics to entertain my friends and family.

My personal favorite party trick is the "sneeze and scream." Basically, I'll start to sneeze and then suddenly let out a blood-curdling scream. It's a guaranteed way to make people jump out of their seats. Of course, it's not so funny when you're in a movie theater and everyone is staring at you like you're a serial killer, but hey, you can't win them all.

Being the center of attention was addictive, and I craved the rush of making people laugh with my tics. I even started to take requests from my classmates, who would ask me to do specific tics for their amusement. "Hey Alina, can you do that one where you scream and then your head spins around like in The Exorcist?" Sure, why not? Let me just summon my inner demon real quick.

But school is a strange time for everyone, especially when you have Tourette's. While my classmates were busy worrying about puberty and crushes, I was more concerned with perfecting my tics and making sure they got the biggest laughs. It was like I had my own comedy club, and I was the star performer.

Of course, there were still those who didn't appreciate my unique brand of humor. The teachers, for example, were not amused when I would interrupt class with a sudden burst of barking or a string of curse words. But hey, if they couldn't handle a little involuntary comedy, then they were clearly in the wrong profession.

Why Fit In When You Can Stand Out?

As I entered my teenage years, I started to realize that my Tourette's was a part of who I was. And you know what? I kind of liked it. Sure, it made me stand out, but that was okay. I mean, who wants to be just like everyone else? Not me, that's for sure.

It was a time when I embraced my Tourette's and turned it into a fashion statement. I mean, who needs a nose ring when you have a tic that makes you look like you're constantly sniffing? I remember the first time I dyed my hair bright pink. My classmates stared at me like I had three heads. But you know what? It was worth it just to see the look on their faces when I started ticking and shouting in the middle of class.

And let's not forget about my punk band. We were terrible, but people loved us. Maybe it was because they knew they could always count on me to scream like a banshee during every performance. Or maybe it was just because we were a bunch of misfits who didn't care what anyone else thought.

Of course, there were times when I felt like I was on display, like a zoo animal or a Kardashian. People would stare at me in public, waiting for me to start ticking. It was like they expected me to perform for them on command. But you know what? I didn't mind. I was happy to oblige.

And then there were the bullies. Oh, the bullies. They thought they could get under my skin by mimicking my tics or calling me names. But little did they know, I had a secret weapon: black humor.

One day, a group of guys started making fun of me in the hallway. They were mocking my tics and calling me all sorts of names. And you know what I did? I walked right up to them and shouted, "You know, I always wanted to be a ventriloquist, but I never had a puppet. Thanks for volunteering!" And then I started tic-talking like a crazy person, throwing my voice all over the place. The guys were so freaked out that they ran away screaming. It was glorious.

I may have been the "Tourette's girl" to some, but to me, I was just Alina, a girl who refused to let her condition define her. And you know what? I think that's what made people like me. I wasn't afraid to be myself, even if it meant shouting the occasional curse word or twitching like a maniac. Because at the end of the day, who wants to be normal? Boring, that's who.

Can't you just stop it?

The Awkward Teenage Years: High School Musical... with Tics

Ah, high school. The land of lockers, lunch lines, and judgmental stares. It's like a breeding ground for insecurity, and if you throw in a dash of Tourette's, it's like adding gasoline to a dumpster fire.

Every day was a new challenge. Would I be able to get through a class without shouting something inappropriate? Would I be able to make it through the cafeteria without spilling my tray everywhere? Spoiler alert: the answer was usually no.

But hey, at least I was never alone. My Tourette's always had my back, making sure I never had to face the humiliation of being the only weird kid in the room. And trust me, there were plenty of other weird kids in high school. Some of them just hid it better than others.

I'll never forget the time I was sitting in history class, trying my best to focus on the lesson, when all of a sudden, my tic decided to kick in. And by "tic," I mean a full-on scream. The whole class turned to stare at me, and I could feel my face turning red with embarrassment. But then something amazing happened. One of the other kids in the class shouted something back at me, like we were having some kind of weird call-and-response conversation. And before I knew it, the whole class was shouting back and forth like we were in some kind of Tourette's choir.

Can't you just stop it?

The Sounds of Silence (And Then Shouting)

High school is the perfect place for anyone looking to hone their skills in social awkwardness. And let me tell you, with Tourette's, I was practically a pro. From the moment I stepped foot in that sea of conformity, I knew I was in trouble.

I mean, come on, who wouldn't want to be friends with the girl who randomly shouts out curse words and twitches like a maniac? I was practically the most popular girl in school. Or at least, that's what I told myself as I ate my lunch alone in the bathroom.

But hey, at least my tics made for some great entertainment. Whenever I felt like things were getting too dull, I'd just let out a loud tic and watch everyone's reactions. It was like my own personal version of Whose Line Is It Anyway, except instead of improv comedy, it was just me shouting "banana" for no reason.

And don't even get me started on the bullies. Oh, they loved to mess with me, but little did they know, I had a secret weapon: my tics. Whenever they tried to push me around, I'd just start shouting out random words until they got so confused they'd forget why they were even picking on me in the first place.

Can't you just stop it?

Sure, high school was a challenge, but I like to think I came out on top. I mean, who needs social skills when you've got tics? And let's be real, who wouldn't want to be friends with the girl who can make you laugh and scare you at the same time?

The Many Uses of Tics

Ah, yes, the beauty of tics – they're not just good for scaring off bullies, they're also great for getting out of things you don't want to do. As a professional ticker, I became quite skilled in using my tics to my advantage.

Need an excuse to skip school? Just let out a loud tic and tell the teacher you need to go to the nurse's office. Need to get out of doing chores at home? Start twitching like a maniac and blame it on your tics. And if you're feeling really creative, you can even use your tics to get out of a bad date. Just start shouting random obscenities and watch your date run for the hills.

Of course, this level of deception isn't for everyone. But when you're a ticker, you learn to adapt to your surroundings. And if that means using your tics to get what you want, so be it. Just don't blame me if you get caught – I can't be held responsible for your lack of tic-tactful finesse.

Can't you just stop it?

Who Needs a Date When You Have Tics?

Ah, teenage romance. A time of awkward fumbling, stolen kisses, and unrequited crushes. For me, it was all of those things... and a whole lot more. Trying to navigate the tricky waters of dating with Tourette's was like trying to steer a ship through a hurricane. Every time I tried to make a move, a tic would pop up and ruin the moment. And if by some miracle I managed to get a date, I'd spend the whole time trying to suppress my tics and failing miserably. But hey, at least it made for some great stories to tell later on.

I remember one time in particular when I was on a date with a guy I really liked. We were sitting in a movie theater, holding hands and trying to watch the film. Everything was going well until I felt the urge to let out a loud tic. I tried to hold it in, but it was no use. Suddenly, I let out a loud bark that echoed throughout the theater. Everyone turned to look at us, and I felt my face turn bright red with embarrassment. But my date just laughed and said, "Well, that's one way to break the ice!" We ended up spending the rest of the day giggling and making tic jokes.

Another time, I had a crush on a guy who was a total jock. He was the star quarterback of the football team, and I was a punk rocker with a penchant for swearing. I knew I didn't stand a chance, but I couldn't help but try. One day, I mustered up the courage to ask him to the school dance. He looked at me like I was crazy and said, "No way, I don't want to catch whatever you've got." I could have been offended, but instead, I just laughed and said, "Trust me, you don't want to catch this tic bug. It's contagious!" He laughed too, and we ended up becoming good friends.

My teenage years were a wild ride of tics, cringe, and mortification. But hey, at least they didn't teach me how to be a boring, conformist drone like everyone else. They taught me to be tough, to own my quirks, and to always keep a sense of humor about it all. And isn't that what being a badass adult is all about?

In Public: Making a Scene and Delighting Strangers

Welcome to the wild and wacky world of public tics. Nothing screams "I'm here and I'm fabulous" like a good tic fit in a crowded room. Whether it's a sudden burst of profanity or a full-body twitch, you're sure to command everyone's attention. And who wouldn't want that, right? Sure, some may stare or whisper behind your back, but that just means you're the talk of the town. So go ahead, let those tics fly and bask in the glory of your uniqueness. Just be prepared for the occasional eye roll or "what the hell?" from the less enlightened individuals. But hey, who needs 'em anyway? You're a public ticker and damn proud of it.

The Art of Making an Entrance

There's nothing quite like the rush of entering a public space and letting your tics run wild. The stares, the gasps, the whispers—it's all part of the thrill. Whether it's the mall, the grocery store, or a crowded street, the possibilities for making an entrance are endless.

I remember one time I went to see a play with my family. As we took our seats, I could feel my tics starting to bubble up inside me. The more I tried to suppress them, the worse they got. And of course, they decided to make their grand entrance during a particularly quiet moment in the play.

As I let out a loud tic, everyone in the theater turned to look at me. I tried to play it off like nothing had happened, but my tics had other ideas. They kept popping up at the worst possible moments, ruining the dramatic tension and causing the other patrons to glare in my direction.

But hey, it wasn't all bad. My tics also had a way of making boring public events more interesting. I remember going to a city council meeting with my mom and dad, expecting it to be a snooze fest. But as soon as I entered the room, my tics started acting up. And you know what? The council members couldn't take their eyes off me. I was like a sideshow attraction, adding some much-needed excitement to an otherwise dull affair.

Can't you just stop it?

The Benefits of Being a Public Ticker

Believe it or not, being a public ticker can actually be a great way to make friends and influence people. People are naturally curious, and tics are a great conversation starter. I've had countless strangers come up to me and ask about my tics, and it's led to some really interesting conversations.

One time I was standing in line at the grocery store, minding my own business, when my tics decided to have a party. My eyes were darting back and forth, my head was twitching, and I was letting out a few choice vocal tics. The woman behind me looked like she was about to run for the hills, so I decided to break the ice.

Sorry about that, I have Tourette's

She relaxed a bit and said, "Oh, that's what that is! I thought you were possessed by a demon or something."

I chuckled, "Yeah, the devil made me do it."

To my surprise, she started laughing too. We ended up chatting for a while about the quirks of Tourette's, and I even managed to teach her a thing or two. By the time we got to the cashier, we were practically best friends. She even gave me a high-five before we parted ways. Who knew that a grocery store tic attack could lead to a new friendship?

One time I was on my way to an important meeting in a taxi when my tics decided to put on a show. My head was jerking, my arms were flailing, and I was letting out a stream of vocal tics that sounded like a Tourette's symphony. The driver was trying his best to ignore me, but it was pretty clear that he was uncomfortable.

"Sorry about that," I said, trying to break the tension. "I have Tourette's."

The driver gave me a nervous smile and said, "Oh, I see. I thought you were having some kind of seizure or something."

I couldn't resist the opportunity for a joke. "Nah, this is just my dance moves. I'm trying to impress you."

The driver actually laughed and we ended up chatting for the rest of the ride, and I even managed to make him forget about the traffic. Who knew that my Tourette's could be such a great icebreaker?

Tic Tock Goes the Clock

Of course, being a public ticker isn't always rainbows and sunshine. There are times when tics can make a social situation awkward or uncomfortable. But hey, that's just part of the package deal.

Once, I attended a fancy dinner party, feeling like a million bucks in my evening gown. As I mingled with the other guests, I tried to suppress my tics, but it was a losing battle.

Suddenly, my tics took over, and I started twitching and shouting uncontrollably. The crystal glasses on the table clinked together, the centerpieces rattled, and the candelabra started swaying dangerously.

Everyone at the table stared at me, horrified. One pompous gentleman in a bowtie piped up, "You really should try to relax, dear. It's all in your head."

I could feel my blood boiling. So, I did what any self-respecting ticker would do. I grabbed my champagne flute and hurled it at the wall, shattering it to pieces. "Oh, really?" I screamed, my tics intensifying. "Maybe you should try to understand that this isn't some nervous tic, but a genuine neurological disorder."

There was a moment of stunned silence before a woman I didn't know burst out laughing. "You're hilarious!" she said, clapping me on the back. "At least someone around here isn't a total snooze-fest."

A few other people joined in, and we even managed to share a few jokes. But the damage had been done. For the rest of the evening, the other guests kept their distance, eyeing me warily.

You know what? I'm not going to apologize for being myself. Did I act out of line? Sure, but when you're dealing with tics, it's not always easy to stay on your best behavior. Maybe next time, I'll just stick to dinner parties with a more relaxed dress code.

In conclusion, being a public ticker is a wild ride. There are ups and downs, but at the end of the day, it's all about embracing who you are and letting your freak flag fly. So the next time you're in a public place and your tics start acting up, just remember: you're not alone, and you're definitely not boring.

Relationships and Tourette's: How to Scare Off Everyone You Meet

Ah, relationships. That wonderful dance of love, compromise, and inevitable disappointment. And when you add Tourette's to the mix? Well, let's just say it's like doing the tango blindfolded with a live porcupine. But fear not, my dear readers, for I am here to guide you through the treacherous waters of dating and relationships with Tourette's.

The Dos and Don'ts of Tourette's Dating

When it comes to dating with Tourette's, there are a few things you need to keep in mind. First of all, be upfront about your tics. Don't wait until the third date to suddenly start barking like a seal or twitching uncontrollably. Trust me, if your potential partner can't handle it? Well, then they're not worth your time anyway.

Another important thing to remember is to find someone who has a good sense of humor. Let's face it, some of our tics can be pretty funny (at least to other people). If you can find someone who can laugh with you and not at you, then you're already halfway there.

I never thought I'd find love, especially with my Tourette's constantly causing chaos in my life. I mean, who would want to be with someone who can't control their own body and shouts random obscenities?

But then, I met Jake. He was kind, understanding, and had a great sense of humor. And, surprisingly enough, he found my tics endearing. He even joked that they made me more interesting than any other girl he had ever met.

Of course, I was hesitant at first. I had been hurt before by people who couldn't handle my tics, and I didn't want to go through that again. But Jake was different. He never made me feel like a freak or an outcast. Instead, he embraced my

Tourette's and made me feel like it was just another part of who I am.

On our first date, I was a ticking time bomb. We went to a posh restaurant, and I was trying to explain my tics while keeping them under control. It was like trying to hold back a tidal wave with a toothpick. As we were chatting, I accidentally jerked my arm, knocking over a glass of red wine all over my dress. Mortified, I apologized profusely, expecting him to be grossed out or angry. But instead, Jake just chuckled and quipped, "Don't worry, it looks like you're wearing a new shade of lipstick." That was when I knew he was a keeper.

As we continued to see each other, I started to open up more about my Tourette's. I told him about all the times it had caused me embarrassment and shame, and he listened without judgment. He even shared some of his own quirks and insecurities with me, making me feel less alone.

But as much as I loved Jake, there was still a part of me that worried about our future together. What if my tics got worse? What if he got tired of dealing with them?

One day, we were walking in the park, and I started ticking uncontrollably. I was shouting and flailing my arms, and I felt so embarrassed. But Jake just put his arms around me and said, "I love you, Alina. All of you. Even the parts that make you tic."

That was when I realized that love isn't about finding someone who's perfect or who can fix all your problems. It's about finding someone who accepts you for who you are, tics and all.

Jake and I have been together for three years now, and my tics have definitely not disappeared. In fact, they've gotten worse at times. But with Jake by my side, I feel like I can handle anything.

We've even started to use my tics as a way to bond and make each other laugh. Sometimes, I'll shout out a random phrase, and Jake will respond with an equally ridiculous one. It's our own little inside joke.

Sure, my Tourette's can still be a challenge at times, but it's also brought me the greatest gift of all: love. And for that, I will always be grateful.

Alright folks, let's talk about what NOT to do when it comes to dating with Tourette's. And let me tell you, the number one don't is trying to hide your tics. Look, I get it, we all want to make a good first impression. But trust me, trying to suppress your tics is a recipe for disaster. Not only is it exhausting, but it's like trying to hold back a sneeze. Eventually, it's gonna come out one way or another, and it's gonna be messy.

Plus, it's not fair to your partner. They deserve to know what they're getting into. It's like ordering a pizza and finding out it has anchovies on it after it's already been delivered. Not cool, man.

And please, for the love of all things holy, don't be ashamed of your tics. They're a part of who you are, like that weird birthmark on your butt. And anyone who can't accept that isn't worth your time. You deserve someone who loves you, tics and all.

Trust me, I've been there. I once went on a date with a guy who was so uptight, I swear he had a stick up his butt. We were at a fancy restaurant, and I ordered a steak. When it arrived, I had a sudden tic and accidentally flung a piece of meat across the table and onto his lap. The worst part? He was wearing white pants. Talk about a stain that's hard to ignore.

I attempted to apologize and clarify that my tic was beyond my control. But guess what this guy did? Zilch. Nada. He just sat there with a face as emotionless as a brick wall, as if he was watching a sloth race. Not a single chuckle or attempt to lighten the mood.

Needless to say, there wasn't a second date. But hey, at least I got a good story out of it. And I learned an important lesson: never suppress your tics for anyone, especially not a guy in white pants.

Can't you just stop it?

So, let your tics fly, my friends. Own them like a boss. Show them off like they're the latest fashion trend. And if someone can't handle it, well, that's their loss. You'll find someone who loves you just the way you are. And if all else fails, there's always pizza.

How to Lose Friends and Alienate People (with Tics)

Let's be honest, Tourette's can be pretty damn off-putting to some people. But you know what? That's their loss. You don't want to waste your time on people who can't handle a little twitching or shouting.

That being said, there are a few things you can do to make sure you're not scaring off potential friends and acquaintances. First of all, try to be aware of your surroundings. If you're in a quiet library or movie theater, maybe hold off on the shouting and twitching for a little while. And if someone does seem uncomfortable with your tics, don't take it personally. It's not a reflection of you as a person.

At the end of the day, having Tourette's can make relationships and friendships a bit more complicated, but it doesn't have to be a dealbreaker. The right people will accept you for who you are, tics and all. And if they don't? Well, then they're not worth your time.

Can't you just stop it?

Just Calm Down: Coping Mechanisms That Don't Work

Ah, coping mechanisms. Those things that people suggest to you with the best intentions, but that always end up being more frustrating than helpful. As someone with Tourette's, I've heard my fair share of coping mechanisms that supposedly help me control my tics. Spoiler alert: most of them don't work. But hey, at least I've got some funny stories to tell about them.

The Many Uses of Deep Breathing (Hint: None of Them Work)

Oh boy, deep breathing. The classic suggestion for relaxation and stress relief. But when you're sitting there in the middle of a tic attack, taking deep breaths is about as useful as wearing a raincoat in a tsunami. I've tried it all, trust me. It's like trying to stop a train with a feather.

One time, I was in a meeting at work and I felt it coming on - the telltale signs of a tic attack brewing in my body. My neck started jerking uncontrollably, and my hand was tapping a mile a minute on the table. I tried to do some deep breathing to calm myself down, but it felt like I was trying to tame a bull with a red cape. Before I knew it, I was yelling random words and barking like a dog. Needless to say, some colleagues were very confused.

I tried to explain to them that it was just my Tourette's acting up. And the worst part? The guy who was leading the meeting just sat there with a blank expression on his face. Not a single chuckle or attempt to lighten the mood. It was like watching paint dry, but less exciting.

I mean, come on. If you can't find the humor in a grown woman barking like a dog in the middle of a meeting, what kind of life are you living? It's not like I was trying to sabotage the company or anything. I just have a neurological

Can't you just stop it?

condition that causes me to make weird noises and movements. It's not like I can help it.

But hey, at least I got to leave the meeting early. And let me tell you, there's nothing quite like stepping out of a room full of people and letting out a string of tics that would make a sailor blush. It's like a pressure valve being released, and for a few blissful moments, I can just be myself without worrying about what other people think.

So yeah, deep breathing may work for some people, but for us Touretters, it's about as useful as a chocolate teapot. Sometimes you just have to let it out, no matter how embarrassing or inappropriate it may seem to others. And if they can't handle it, well, that's their problem.

Meditation? More Like Aggravation

Ah, meditation. The ultimate battle between inner peace and uncontrollable tics. It's like trying to herd cats, only the cats are shouting and twitching and you're the crazy one in the corner trying to meditate. I mean, come on, who needs quiet and serenity when you can have your own personal symphony of tics, am I right?

I've attempted to meditate in the past, but it always ends up being an exercise in futility. Trying to calm my mind only makes my tics even louder, like they're saying "Oh, you thought you could forget about us for a minute? Think again!" It's like trying to relax in the middle of a metal concert - not gonna happen.

One time, I thought I'd give it a shot in a yoga class. I mean, isn't yoga supposed to be all about finding inner peace and harmony? Well, let me tell you, my tics had other plans. As soon as the instructor suggested we meditate, my tics went into overdrive. Shouting, twitching, the whole nine yards. I'm pretty sure I ruined everyone's zen that day. Namaste, my ass.

So, if you're like me and your tics refuse to take a break, just embrace them. Maybe you can turn them into a new form of meditation. Call it "Ticitation" or something. Who needs the sound of the ocean when you can have the sound of your own personal tics? Just be sure to warn your fellow yogis first.

Why Run When You Can Twitch?

Now this is a coping mechanism I can get behind. Instead of trying to fight my tics or suppress them, I've learned to embrace them. And you know what? It's actually kind of liberating. Instead of feeling ashamed or embarrassed about my tics, I've started using them to my advantage. For example, if I'm in a boring meeting or conversation, I'll let my tics out a little bit to keep myself entertained. It's like having my own personal entertainment system built right in.

Who needs regular hobbies when you can turn your own body into a non-stop source of entertainment? It's like being a human version of those wind-up toys that bounce all over the place. Now, when I feel a tic attack coming on, I don't panic - I get excited. What kind of crazy tic is going to come out next? Will I shout out a random word? Will I start twerking? The possibilities are endless!

I've found that embracing my tics has also been a great way to weed out people who can't handle a little spontaneity. If I'm on a date and the person can't handle me randomly blurting out "ridiculous underpants," then he's probably not the one for me. It's like a built-in compatibility test. And let's be real, anyone who can't handle a little tics-induced humor isn't worth my time anyway.

Of course, there are some downsides to this approach. Like when I'm trying to have a serious conversation and my tics decide it's time for a dance party. Or when I'm in a library and I accidentally scream out "SHHHHHH!" But hey, no one said living with Tourette's was easy. At least I can find the humor in it all.

In conclusion, coping mechanisms can be helpful for some people, but for those of us with Tourette's, they can often be more frustrating than anything else. Instead of trying to fight our tics or suppress them, we should embrace them and use them to our advantage. After all, who needs deep breathing when you can just let out a good tic?

Can't you just stop it?

Tics in the Workplace: How to Get Fired in 10 Seconds or Less

Ah, the workplace. A place of productivity, professionalism, and plenty of opportunities to embarrass yourself with a well-timed tic. As someone with Tourette's, I know all too well the challenges of working in a professional environment. Let's dive into the world of tics in the workplace, shall we?

Can't you just stop it?

Office Life with Tourette's

The first challenge of working with Tourette's is finding a workplace that accommodates your tics. Unfortunately, not all workplaces are created equal. Some are more understanding than others. In my experience, smaller companies are often more accommodating than larger ones. I once worked for a large corporation that had no idea how to handle my tics. They suggested I wear a mask to cover my face tics. Yeah, because that wouldn't draw attention to me at all.

Another challenge is dealing with coworkers who don't understand Tourette's. I've lost count of how many times I've been asked if I'm okay, if I need medical attention, or if I'm possessed by a demon. Yes, because that's exactly what I want to hear when I'm trying to focus on work.

And let's not forget about the joys of open-concept offices. You know, the ones where everyone can see and hear everything you do. I once worked in an office like this and my tics were so distracting that my coworkers started betting on what my next tic would be. I'm pretty sure I was the most entertaining thing in the office.

Can't you just stop it?

My Boss Hates Me

Well, ain't that just a barrel of laughs. Nothing like being discriminated against for something that's completely out of your control. I once had a boss who thought my tics were a sign that I was possessed by demons. I mean, come on, at least make it interesting - I'd rather be possessed by a demon than have Tourette's.

But discrimination doesn't just come from the higher-ups. Oh no, your lovely coworkers can get in on the fun too. I once had a coworker who complained to HR about my tics because she thought they were "disruptive" and "unprofessional". Well, excuse me, Karen, for not being able to control my involuntary muscle movements while I'm trying to do my job. Maybe you should take a break from your Pinterest board and educate yourself on Tourette's instead.

And let's not forget the classic move of not being given important tasks because of your tics. Because clearly, my ability to get things done is directly correlated to my twitching and shouting. I mean, I get it, it's not like I have a college degree or years of experience in my field. Nope, it's all about the tics.

But hey, at least we can always rely on HR to have our backs, right? Wrong. I once had an HR representative ask me if I could just "stop doing the tic thing" during important meetings. Oh sure, let me just turn off my neurological

Can't you just stop it?

disorder like a light switch, that'll be easy. Thanks for the helpful suggestion, Brenda.

All in all, navigating the workplace with Tourette's can be a real barrel of laughs. But hey, at least we can all laugh about it, right? Hahaha, oh wait, no we can't, because our tics make us look like we're having a seizure.

Tourette's and HR

Speaking of HR, let's talk about how to file a complaint when you're experiencing discrimination or harassment in the workplace. The first step is to document everything. Keep a record of any comments or actions that are discriminatory or harassing. This will be important evidence if you need to take further action.

The second step is to approach HR with your concerns. Be clear and concise about what's been happening and how it's affecting you. Be prepared to offer solutions or suggestions for how the situation can be improved. And don't forget to advocate for yourself - you deserve to be treated with respect and dignity in the workplace.

Of course, filing a complaint can be a risky move. It's important to consider the potential consequences and how they might affect your job. Will HR actually do something about it or just give you a pat on the back and a "thanks for letting us know"? And let's not forget about the potential retaliation from your boss or coworkers. Suddenly you're the outcast of the office, eating lunch alone and wondering if you'll ever feel the sweet embrace of normalcy again. So go ahead, spin that complaint chamber and see what happens - just don't be surprised if it backfires in your face.

Living with Tourette's can be like trying to find a needle in a haystack - it's hard to find a workplace that won't make you feel like a circus act. People can be so ignorant and discriminatory that it's a wonder they can even tie their own shoes. But fear not, my fellow tic-ridden comrades! With a little bit of advocacy and a whole lot of patience, you can find a workplace that won't make you want to scream your head off. So keep your chin up, keep your tics in check, and keep on looking - because there's a job out there for all of us freaks.

The Humor in Tics: Laughing Through the Pain and Discomfort

Life with Tourette's can be a real rollercoaster ride. One minute you're laughing at your tics, and the next you're sobbing into a pillow because you just can't control your body. But that's where humor comes in handy. It's like a safety net for those moments when you feel like you're about to fall off the crazy train. So go ahead and embrace the absurdity of it all, because sometimes the only thing left to do is laugh.

Can't you just stop it?

Tourette's as a Comedy Goldmine

As someone with Tourette's, I have a lot of experience with awkward and embarrassing situations. But you know what they say, laughter is the best medicine, and I've found that finding the humor in these situations can make them a lot less painful.

For example, I once had a tic where I would make a very loud and very distinct quacking noise. It was especially embarrassing when it happened in quiet places, like during a movie or in a library. But one day, I decided to lean into it and started quacking every time someone said something that I found particularly ridiculous. Soon, my friends started catching on and we turned it into a game. It was like our own little inside joke, and it made me feel a lot less self-conscious about my tic.

Of course, not everyone is going to find humor in their tics, and that's okay. But for those of us who do, it can be a great coping mechanism.

"Tic Talk": Inside Jokes and Tic-Specific Humor

As I mentioned earlier, finding humor in your tics can be a great way to cope with them. But sometimes, that humor can be even more specific. Tic-specific humor, if you will.

For example, there are some tics that are just so ridiculous that you can't help but laugh at them. Like when I have a tic where I have to shake my head really hard and fast. It looks like I'm trying to shake off water like a dog. And the reactions I get from people are priceless. I've seen grown men jump out of their seats and spill their coffee all over themselves because of that tic. It's pure entertainment.

Having a friend who shares your tics is priceless. There's nothing like bonding over involuntary movements and strange noises. My friend Omar and I both have Tourette's, and we share a hilarious inside joke. You see, we both have a tic where we make a screeching noise that sounds like a pterodactyl. Yes, you read that right, a pterodactyl! It's like we're living in the Jurassic era, but with less danger and more laughter. And let me tell you, nothing beats the feeling of being able to make a ridiculous noise and having your friend understand and join in on the fun. It's like our own little secret language, and it's one of the many reasons why having Tourette's can be both challenging and hilarious at the same time.

Can't you just stop it?

The Joy of Swearing

Okay, let's be real. One of the most famous things about Tourette's is the swearing. And while not everyone with Tourette's has a swearing tic, those of us who do know that it can be pretty hilarious.

I personally have a tic where I yell out "Oh, for f***'s sake!" at random intervals. And while it can be embarrassing in certain situations, I have to admit, there's something satisfying about being able to curse like a sailor without anyone batting an eye.

Of course, it's important to be mindful of where and when you swear, especially if you're around children or in a professional setting. But when you're with friends who understand your tics, there's nothing quite like being able to let loose and say exactly what you're thinking, no matter how foul-mouthed it may be.

So there you have it, folks. The joys of humor and tics. Because when life gives you involuntary movements and vocalizations, sometimes the only thing you can do is laugh.

Can't you just stop it?

Fighting Stigma: How to Convince People You're Not Possessed by the Devil

Stigma, or the bane of my existence! If there's one thing I've learned from living with Tourette's syndrome, it's that people can be pretty ignorant. And let me tell you, nothing is more fun than trying to convince someone that I'm not possessed by the devil or just trying to get attention.

So let's dive into this chapter on fighting stigma and try to educate the masses.

Tourette's: More Than Just Tics

The classic misconception that Tourette's is just about yelling curse words and twitching. It's as if people think I'm starring in my own personal episode of The Exorcist. But let me tell you, there's so much more to it than that.

For starters, Tourette's is a neurological disorder that affects much more than just my motor and vocal tics. It can cause anxiety, depression, and OCD-like symptoms, just to name a few. And while my tics might be the most noticeable aspect of my disorder, they're just the tip of the iceberg.

Another common myth is that Tourette's is caused by bad parenting or a lack of discipline. I mean, why else would a kid be swearing and twitching all over the place, right? Wrong. Tourette's is a genetic disorder that I inherited from my parents. So if you really want to blame someone for my tics, blame my DNA.

No, I'm Not Faking It

Oh boy, this is a fun one. Nothing like being accused of faking a neurological disorder. As if I have nothing better to do than pretend to have uncontrollable tics that make me look like a complete weirdo in public.

Can't you just stop it?

But sadly, skepticism is all too common when it comes to Tourette's. I've had people tell me that I'm just seeking attention, or that I could stop my tics if I really wanted to. And let me tell you, nothing is more frustrating than trying to explain to someone that I literally cannot control my tics.

But hey, I try to have a sense of humor about it. Once, a guy at a party asked me if I could stop ticking if he gave me $20. I told him that if he gave me $20, I'd be able to tic louder. He didn't find it as funny as I did.

The Everyday Struggle

At the end of the day, living with Tourette's can be exhausting. It's hard enough dealing with the physical and emotional toll of my tics, but on top of that, I have to deal with people's ignorance and skepticism.

It's not easy being different, and sometimes I just wish I could blend in with the crowd. But at the same time, I know that my Tourette's has shaped me into the person I am today. It's taught me empathy, resilience, and a whole lot of patience.

And hey, it's not all bad. Sometimes my tics can be pretty funny, even to me. Like the time I was at a quiet library and my tic made me shout "I LIKE PICKLES!" at the top of my lungs. The librarian was not amused, but I couldn't stop laughing.

So to anyone out there who's struggling with Tourette's or any other disorder that makes them feel different, know that you're not alone. And hey, maybe one day we'll live in a world where people don't judge us for things that are out of our control. But until then, we'll just keep on ticking.

Can't you just stop it?

Twitching Through the Globe: My Tourettes-infused Travel Diaries

Ah, the joys of travel with Tourette's! As if dealing with cramped airplane seats and lost luggage isn't enough, try explaining to customs why you can't stop twitching and shouting. But fear not, my fellow Touretters, I've got you covered.

Dealing with Customs

As if the usual questioning and bag checks weren't enough, now you have to explain why you're twitching and shouting like a madman. My go-to line is "I have Tourette's," but sometimes they'll want proof. That's when I bust out my handy-dandy medical alert bracelet or doctor's note. But if you really want to have some fun, try telling them you're smuggling rare bird calls in your vocal tics.

One time, I was going through customs in a foreign country and the officer was giving me the stink eye. He asked me why I was twitching so much and I replied, "Oh, I'm just doing my impression of a malfunctioning robot. Beep boop." He didn't seem amused, but luckily my doctor's note got me through without any issues.

Another time, I was traveling with a group of friends and we were all going through customs together. As we were waiting in line, I couldn't help but tic out "I have Tourette's" in a high-pitched voice. My friend next to me, quick on his feet, turned to the customs officer and said, "Oh don't mind her, she's just really excited to be here." The officer just gave us a bewildered look and let us through.

But the best customs story I have is when I was traveling with my family and we were going through security. My tics were particularly bad that day and I was having trouble keeping my hands still. The security officer asked me if I had anything in my pockets and I blurted out "No, just my hands doing their own thing." My mom, not missing a beat, added "Yeah, her hands are really independent." The officer just rolled his eyes and waved us through.

At the end of the day, dealing with customs can be a pain, but sometimes a little humor can go a long way.

Making Friends in Foreign Lands

Making friends in foreign lands can be a challenge, especially when you're constantly twitching and making weird noises. But fear not, my fellow Touretters, because I've got some tips and tricks up my sleeve.

First off, embrace the culture. If you're in Italy, throw in some hand gestures with your tics and pretend you're just being extra expressive in the Italian way. If you're in Japan, bow your head as part of your tics and convince them that it's a sign of respect. The possibilities are endless, really.

Another trick is to play up the comedic aspect of your tics. People love a good laugh, so if you can make your tics seem like part of a stand-up routine, they'll be more likely to embrace you. I once had a tic that made me flap my arms like a chicken, and I turned it into a hilarious dance move that had everyone in stitches.

And if all else fails, just blame it on your country's stereotype. For example, if you're American, tell people that your tics are just a result of growing up on too much fast food and reality TV. They'll either laugh and nod in agreement or just assume that all Americans are crazy.

But really, the key to making friends with your tics is just to be yourself. Embrace your quirks and don't be afraid to show them off. People are more likely to accept you when you're confident in who you are. And who knows, maybe your tics will even become a conversation starter and lead to some amazing friendships.

Tourist Attractions with Tics

Let me tell you about my experience seeing the world one twitch at a time. When I visited the Great Wall of China, I couldn't resist doing a little hop and skip every few steps. And when I finally reached the top, my tics kicked into overdrive with some extra loud "woohoo's" and fist pumps. It definitely added a little extra excitement to the experience.

And let's not forget about visiting museums and galleries. Sure, you could appreciate the art in silence like a "normal" person, but where's the fun in that? I like to spice things up by throwing in some vocal tics or interpretive dance moves. The confused looks from other patrons just add to the entertainment value.

Can't you just stop it?

And let's not forget about amusement parks. Rollercoasters and other thrill rides are already a rush, but throw in some tics and it's a whole new level of excitement. I remember going on a ride that had a loop and every time we went upside down, I couldn't resist yelling "Whee!" at the top of my lungs. The people in the car with me were a little taken aback, but hey, they'll never forget that ride.

So, don't be afraid to embrace your tics and incorporate them into your travels. You never know what kind of fun and memorable experiences they'll lead to. Just be prepared for some curious looks and questions from fellow travelers.

How to Say "I Have Tourettes" in Every Language

As someone with Tourette's, I've had my fair share of language barriers while traveling. It's not easy trying to explain to someone that you're not speaking in tongues, you just have an involuntary tic disorder. That's why I've made it my personal mission to learn how to say "I have Tourette's" in every language I might encounter on my travels.

It's not always easy to find the right words, especially when you're dealing with tonal languages like Mandarin or Thai. But with a little practice and a lot of patience, I've managed to master the basics. And let me tell you, there's nothing quite like the look on someone's face when you drop a perfectly accented "J'ai le syndrome de Gilles de la Tourette" in the middle of a French café.

But it's not just about impressing the locals with your linguistic skills. Knowing how to say "I have Tourette's" can also be a lifesaver in certain situations. Take the time I was traveling through a particularly sketchy part of Costa Rica. I was surrounded by a group of men who were shouting at me in Spanish, and my tics were going into overdrive. I managed to blurt out "Tengo el síndrome de Tourette" just in time for them to back off and give me some space.

Of course, not every encounter is quite so dramatic. Sometimes it's just a matter of explaining to your waiter why you keep shouting "I'll have what she's having" every time you see someone else's food go by. Or reassuring the person next to you on the train that you're not having some kind of seizure, you're just twitchy.

And let's not forget the fun of trying to communicate with locals who don't speak any of the languages you've mastered. That's when you break out the international language of charades. Want to explain to your new friends in Tokyo that you're not insulting them, you're just trying to suppress a vocal tic? Just start miming a karaoke performance and hope for the best.

At the end of the day, language barriers are just one more obstacle for those of us with Tourette's to navigate while traveling. But with a little creativity and a lot of humor, we can turn those obstacles into opportunities for connection and understanding.

Support Groups: Because You're Not the Only One Freaking Out

Alright, let's talk about support groups. No, not the kind where you hold hands and sing Kumbaya, but the kind where you gather with other people who also can't control their twitches and tics. It's like a family reunion, only instead of discussing your aunt's weird potato salad, you're talking about your Tourettesy struggles. And let me tell you, it's a real hoot. Because when you're surrounded by people who get it, suddenly your tics and twitches become a source of entertainment. It's like a comedy show, but instead of paying for a ticket, you're paying with your sanity. But hey, at least you're not alone in this crazy Tourettesy world.

The Joy of Being the Most Tourettesy Person in the Room

There's nothing quite like walking into a support group and realizing that, for once, you're not the only one who's constantly twitching and vocalizing. It's like being a celebrity - everyone's eyes are on you, wondering what kind of crazy tic you'll bust out next.

As soon as I enter the support group, I feel like I'm in my element. It's a place where I can let my tics run wild without fear of judgment. I take a deep breath and let out a loud bark, and suddenly, all eyes are on me. It's a rush, like I'm the star of my own little show. And the best part is, I don't have to explain myself or feel self-conscious. In fact, the more outrageous my tics, the more impressed people seem to be. It's like I'm a Tourette's savant, and everyone else is just trying to keep up. So yeah, call me crazy, but there's a certain joy in being the most Tourettesy person in the room. It's like being part of a secret club where the only requirement is a tendency to twitch and make strange noises. And who wouldn't want to be part of that club?

Can't you just stop it?

Sharing is Caring

Support groups can be a real lifesaver for those of us with Tourette's. It's a chance to connect with others who understand what it's like to constantly be twitching and vocalizing. But let's be honest, the best part of these support groups is the opportunity to share stories about our weirdest tics.

It's like a Tourette's version of show and tell. You walk into the room, and everyone's eyes are on you, waiting to see what kind of crazy tic you'll bust out next. It's like being a magician, but instead of pulling a rabbit out of a hat, you're pulling out a spontaneous burst of vocalizations.

And the stories that get shared in these groups? Let me tell you, they're gold. One person will talk about how they involuntarily bark like a dog, and then someone else will chime in about their tic that involves randomly meowing like a cat. It's like a never-ending game of one-upmanship.

But it's not just about the hilarity of it all. Sharing stories about our tics is a way to connect with others and feel less alone. It's a reminder that we're not the only ones dealing with this condition, and that there are others out there who understand what it's like.

And let's be real, sometimes these stories are just downright ridiculous. I once heard about someone who had a tic that involved pretending to be a flamingo. Yes, you read that right. They would stand on one leg, flap their arms, and make squawking noises. And you know what? We all laughed about it. Because when everyone in the room is twitching and vocalizing, everything's hilarious.

But it's not just about laughing at each other's tics. It's about finding the humor in our own condition and learning to embrace it. Tourette's can be a frustrating and isolating experience, but it doesn't have to be all doom and gloom. Sometimes, all it takes is a good laugh to help us see things in a different light.

And let's be real, sometimes our tics can be pretty darn entertaining. I mean, who wouldn't want to see someone randomly start clucking like a chicken in the middle of a support group meeting? It's like a built-in comedy routine.

The Power of Laughter

Support groups for Tourettes can be a barrel of laughs. When you're in a room full of people who all understand what it's like to have Tourettes, everything suddenly becomes hilarious. One person starts ticking, and soon everyone else is joining in, and before you know it, you're all in tears from laughing so hard. It's like a contagious laughter that spreads from one person to the other. Who needs a comedy club when you've got a support group? And let's be real, sometimes the tics themselves are just plain funny. Whether it's a sudden outburst of a random phrase or a spontaneous dance move, when everyone in the room is twitching, everything's hilarious. And the best part? You don't have to worry about anyone judging you for your tics, because they're all in the same boat. So let loose and let the laughter flow.

But all joking aside, sharing stories about our tics is an important part of coping with Tourette's. It's a way to connect with others and remind ourselves that we're not alone in this. And if we can find a way to laugh about it all, even better. Because when it comes down to it, sometimes the best medicine is just a good old-fashioned belly laugh.

Can't you just stop it?

Navigating the Medical System: Where They Make You Feel Crazy for Being Tourettesy

Navigating the medical system as a Touretter is like playing a game of hide-and-seek, only you're the one hiding from doctors who have no clue what to do with you. You find yourself in a room with a stranger in a white coat who's asking you questions that seem to have nothing to do with your tics, while you silently wonder if you've accidentally walked into a job interview. And then there's the added bonus of being told to "just relax" or "stop thinking about it so much," as if your tics are just a figment of your imagination.

Doctor Knows Best... or Not

Ah, the joys of being misdiagnosed by doctors who are convinced that your tics must be caused by some other underlying issue. "It's just stress," they'll say, as if you haven't already tried every stress-relief technique known to man. Or even better, when they try to attribute your tics to some obscure disease that they just learned about in med school. Sorry, Doc, but I don't think my Tourettes is caused by a rare tropical fungus.

But don't worry, my fellow Touretters, because we're strong and we know how to advocate for ourselves. We know when something's not right, and we're not afraid to speak up and demand the proper care and treatment. And when we finally find a doctor who truly understands Tourettes and listens to us, it's like finding a unicorn. Cherish them, my friends, for they are a rare and precious breed.

And let's not forget about the endless referrals to specialists who have no idea how to treat Tourettes. You'll get sent to a neurologist who specializes in Parkinson's disease, a psychiatrist who thinks your tics are caused by some deep-seated trauma, and a physical therapist who's convinced that you just need some exercise to make those tics go away. It's like a game of medical roulette, and you never know what kind of doctor you'll end up with next.

Can't you just stop it?

But despite the frustration of navigating the medical system, we Touretters are a resilient bunch. We know what we need, and we won't stop until we get it. We'll fight tooth and nail to get the treatments and accommodations we deserve, and we won't let anyone tell us that our tics aren't real or that we're just making them up for attention. So bring on the doctors, bring on the specialists, and bring on the misdiagnoses. We're ready for anything that the medical system can throw at us.

In the end, we're the ones who know our Tourettes best. We live with it every day, and we know exactly what we need to manage our symptoms and live our best lives. So don't be afraid to speak up and advocate for yourself in the medical system. You are your own best advocate, and no one knows your Tourettes better than you do.

Insurance Woes

And then there's the issue of insurance. It's like a never-ending cycle of frustration. You need treatment for your Tourettes, but your insurance won't cover it unless you jump through a million hoops. And when you finally manage to jump through all those hoops, they just add a few more for good measure. It's like they're trying to see just how much you're willing to put up with. But hey, at least you're getting a good workout from all that jumping.

And let's not forget about the joy of pre-authorization. You know, that wonderful process where you have to prove to your insurance company that you actually need the treatment they're denying you. Because clearly, they know your body better than you do. And if you're lucky enough to get approved, don't get too excited. There's always the chance that your insurance company will suddenly decide they don't want to cover it anymore and leave you high and dry.

And don't even get me started on the cost of medication. Who needs a savings account when you can just pay for your medication with your first-born child, right? And of course, those meds come with a whole host of side effects that make you wonder if they're really worth it. But hey, at least you'll have a good excuse for any sudden weight gain or uncontrollable flatulence.

But all joking aside, fighting with insurance companies can be exhausting and demoralizing. It's a constant battle to get the treatment you need and deserve. And unfortunately, not everyone has the privilege of being able to afford it without insurance. It's a broken system, but we have to keep fighting. We have to keep advocating for ourselves and for others who may not have the same resources or support. And in the meantime, we can at least try to find some humor in the absurdity of it all. After all, laughter is the best medicine...unless you can't afford it.

Can't you just stop it?

Medication Frustration

Last but not least, there's the never-ending battle of finding the right medication balance. It's like Goldilocks and the Three Bears, except instead of porridge, it's pills. One makes you too tired, one makes you too jittery, and one makes you feel like a zombie.

Tourette's medication is like playing Russian roulette with your brain, except the bullets are pills and the gun is your body. You never know which pill is going to make you feel like you just chugged a whole pot of coffee or like you've been hit by a tranquilizer dart. And let's not forget the delightful side effects that come with each medication. One makes you gain weight faster than a competitive eater, while another makes you so gassy you could power a hot air balloon. It's like the pharmaceutical companies saw how much we were struggling with Tourette's and decided to throw in a free circus act with every prescription. But hey, at least we're keeping things interesting, right?

But let's not forget the bright side of all this medication madness: the quest for the perfect balance. It's like being a mad scientist in your own body, except instead of creating a monster, you're just trying to function like a regular human being. It's a delicate dance of trial and error, but when you finally find that perfect pill cocktail, it's like the clouds part and the sun shines down upon you. Suddenly, you're able to do things you never thought possible, like sit still for an entire movie or hold a conversation without any interruptions. It's like hitting the Tourettes jackpot. And by jackpot, I mean being able to go a full five minutes without a tic. Victory.

But even when you do find that perfect medication balance, it's not always smooth sailing. There are still the occasional hiccups, like when your insurance decides to stop covering your medication for no apparent reason. It's like playing a game of chess, except the insurance company is playing with your mental health and the stakes are way higher than just a fancy trophy. But don't worry, you can always appeal their decision and hope that someone on the other end is feeling generous that day. It's like playing the lottery, except instead of money, you could win the right to keep taking the medication that keeps you functioning like a semi-normal human being.

So, in the end, Tourette's medication may be a frustrating and expensive rollercoaster ride, but at least it keeps life interesting. It's like the cherry on top of an already complicated sundae. And hey, if all else fails, you can always just embrace your tics and turn them into a party trick.

Life Lessons: How Tourette's Has Made Me a Better Human Being (Just Kidding)

Oh boy, a chapter about how Tourette's has made me a better person. This is going to be a real tearjerker. Just kidding, I'm not that sentimental. But let's explore how Tourette's has supposedly made me a better human being, shall we?

Tourette's and Empathy

As someone who has lived with Tourette's for most of my life, I can attest to the fact that it has taught me a great deal about what it's like to live with a condition that affects every aspect of your life.

When you have Tourette's, you quickly learn that not everyone is going to understand or accept your condition. You might encounter people who stare at you or make fun of your tics, or even those who discriminate against you in the workplace or school. These experiences can be incredibly isolating, and they can make you feel like no one else truly understands what you're going through.

But as you begin to connect with others who are dealing with chronic diseases, you realize that you're not alone in your struggles. You start to see that everyone has their own challenges and obstacles to overcome, and that the best way to get through them is to support and uplift one another.

For me, this realization came when I met someone who had Parkinson's disease. Although our conditions were different, we were both dealing with the reality of having a condition that made us stand out and that affected our ability to do certain things. When we started talking about our experiences, we both realized how much we had in common. We both knew what it was like to feel misunderstood, and we both knew the importance of finding supportive people who could help us through our toughest moments.

This connection with someone who was dealing with a different chronic disease helped me to develop a sense of empathy that I don't think I would have otherwise had. I began to see that the struggles that I was going through were not unique to me, and that there were countless other people out there who were dealing with similar challenges. This realization helped me to become more patient and understanding with others, and it taught me the importance of supporting those who might be going through a tough time.

Of course, developing empathy is not something that happens overnight. It takes time and effort to truly understand what others are going through, and it requires a willingness to listen and learn from others. But I truly believe that having Tourette's can help set you on the path towards developing empathy, as it forces you to confront the reality of living with a chronic condition.

So, if you're living with Tourette's or any other chronic disease, know that you're not alone in your struggles. There are countless others out there who are dealing with similar challenges, and who can help you develop a greater sense of empathy and understanding. Whether you connect with others through support groups, online forums, or just by reaching out to those around you, know that there is strength in numbers and that you can make a positive difference in the lives of others.

In the Face of Adversity

Apparently, Tourette's makes you more resilient and adaptable. Well, color me surprised. I never realized that constant twitching and involuntary noises made me the poster child for adaptability.

Sure, I've developed some coping mechanisms over the years to deal with my tics, but let's not get carried away here. It's not like I suddenly turned into a superhero with a cape made out of tic repellent. I still have days where I feel like throwing in the towel and giving up altogether. And don't even get me started on the anxiety and frustration that comes with having particularly bad tics.

Honestly, I'm not sure how much resilience and adaptability you can really develop when you're constantly at war with your own body. It's like trying to win a game of tug-of-war with a bulldozer. Yeah, good luck with that.

But hey, at least I can say that I've learned to adapt to a life of constantly being stared at and judged by others. I mean, who needs privacy and dignity when you can have a crowd of strangers gawking at you like you're a sideshow attraction? And let's not forget about the joy of explaining your tics to every new person you meet. Nothing like a good ol' game of 20 questions to start off a new friendship.

In all seriousness though, I do believe that having Tourette's has forced me to become more adaptable in some ways. It's taught me to be more patient, understanding, and compassionate towards others who are struggling with their own chronic conditions. And let's face it, there's nothing quite like having a condition that most people don't understand to make you more empathetic towards others.

But let's not pretend that having Tourette's is some kind of magic recipe for resilience and adaptability. It's a constant battle that takes a toll on both your physical and mental health. So, if you'll excuse me, I'm going to go have a good cry and then maybe, just maybe, I'll find the strength to keep on ticking.

The Silver Lining

Well, I guess you could say that Tourette's has given me the gift of being able to laugh at myself. Not in the "I'm so hilarious, everyone should be laughing at me" kind of way, but in the "well, at least I'm not boring" kind of way. I mean, let's face it, I'm pretty unique with my involuntary noises and movements. But instead of feeling ashamed or embarrassed about it, I've learned to embrace my differences and find the humor in the situation.

Can't you just stop it?

It's kind of like when you trip and fall in front of a crowd of people. Sure, it's embarrassing in the moment, but once you get up and realize you're okay, you can laugh at yourself and move on. Same goes for my Tourette's tics. They might seem weird and uncomfortable in the moment, but once I'm past it, I can chuckle about it and move on.

Plus, being able to laugh at myself has made me more approachable and relatable to others. It's like saying, "hey, I might be different, but I'm still human and I can still have a good time." It's a valuable lesson that I wouldn't have learned if it weren't for my Tourette's.

So, to all my fellow Tourette's comrades out there, don't be afraid to embrace your quirks and find the humor in your tics. Life's too short to take ourselves too seriously.

Tic, Tock, Don't Mock!

And finally, this is for any person who thinks it's appropriate to add "comedian" to their resume just because they can make fun of my Tourette's: you must have a pretty boring life if you have nothing better to do than mock someone for something they can't control. Seriously, go find a hobby or something.

I get it, my tics can be weird and unexpected, but that doesn't give you a free pass to make me the punchline of your joke. I'm not a clown here for your entertainment. I'm a person with feelings, emotions, and struggles, just like you. The only difference is that my struggles happen to manifest in the form of tics and involuntary movements.

And while you may find it amusing to imitate me or make sarcastic comments about my condition, I can guarantee you that it's not so funny when you're the one dealing with Tourette's. Imagine having to constantly worry about embarrassing yourself in public or being ridiculed by others. It's not exactly a walk in the park.

So, the next time you feel the urge to make fun of someone with Tourette's, take a step back and ask yourself: is this really worth it? Is my fleeting moment of amusement worth potentially hurting someone else's feelings and perpetuating ignorance about a serious neurological condition?

Can't you just stop it?

If the answer is yes, then go ahead, keep making your little jokes and imitations. Keep pretending like you're so clever and superior. But just know that while you're laughing at me, everyone else is laughing at you. Because let's face it, there's nothing more pathetic than someone who feels the need to put down others to make themselves feel better.

And if the answer is no, then congratulations, you're one step closer to being a decent human being. But hey, maybe I should thank you. After all, dealing with your constant mockery has given me a thick skin and a killer sense of humor.

Can't you just stop it?

My Tourette's Story Ends... or Does It?

Well, it looks like we've reached the end of Tic Talk. What a wild ride it's been! From the early days of my tics to navigating relationships and the workplace, it's been a journey full of surprises, challenges, and plenty of laughs.

Looking back, it's hard to believe how much I've learned about myself and others along the way. I've discovered coping mechanisms that don't work (looking at you, deep breathing), embraced the humor in my tics, and even found a way to turn the tables on stigma and misconceptions. Who knew having Tourette's could be so entertaining?

But let's not forget that living with tics isn't always easy. It can be exhausting, frustrating, and isolating. It can make us feel like outsiders in a world that doesn't always understand us. But through it all, we've developed resilience, empathy, and a unique perspective on life. And hey, if nothing else, at least we can entertain the masses with our random outbursts and movements.

As I close the book on my Tourette's journey, I can't help but wonder what the future holds. Will my tics continue to surprise me? Will I find new ways to navigate the challenges that come my way? One thing's for sure: I'll always have a sense of humor about it all. After all, laughter truly is the best medicine (except for maybe some medication to help with the tics).

Can't you just stop it?

So here's to all the tickers out there, laughing through the pain and discomfort. Keep on twitching and shouting, my friends. Who knows what kind of adventures await us next?

Can't you just stop it?

www.ingramcontent.com/pod-product-compliance
Lightning Source LLC
Chambersburg PA
CBHW061616250726
48653CB00016B/2264